SELF-HELP FOR H

A naturopathic pra ... es of this distressing ailment and its succe ... g a programme of self-help Nature Cure principles.

By the same author:
DIETS TO HELP COLITIS

Self-Help for Hiatus Hernia

Joan Lay N.D., M.B.N.O.A.

THORSONS PUBLISHERS LIMITED
Wellingborough, Northamptonshire

First published 1982
Seventh Impression 1985

British Library Cataloguing in Publication Data

Lay, Joan
Self-help for hiatus hernia.
1. Hiatal hernia 2. Self-care, Health
I. Title
616.3'2 RD621

ISBN 0-7225-0713-5

Printed in Great Britain by
Richard Clay (The Chaucer Press) Ltd,
Bungay, Suffolk

Contents

1.
What Is Hiatus Hernia?

The medical definition of hiatus hernia is: 'displacement of a portion of the stomach through the opening in the diaphragm through which the oesophagus passes from the chest to the abdominal cavity.' To put it another way: a part of the upper wall of the stomach protrudes through the diaphragm at the point where the gullet passes from the chest area to the abdominal area.

The diaphragm is a large dome-shaped muscle, dividing the chest from the abdominal cavity. It is the muscle concerned with breathing, and it is assisted by the intercostal muscles (those between the ribs) during exertion. It has special openings in it to allow for the passage of important blood vessels (the aorta and the vena cava) and for the food channel (the oesophagus). It is the oesophageal opening (hiatus) that concerns us here, because this is the point where the hernia occurs.

Such hernias become increasingly common after middle age, and it is said that about half the population of over sixty years of age suffers from them, although often without any symptoms. A barium x-ray is required for

Diaphragm seen from below, showing the openings and extent of the muscle.

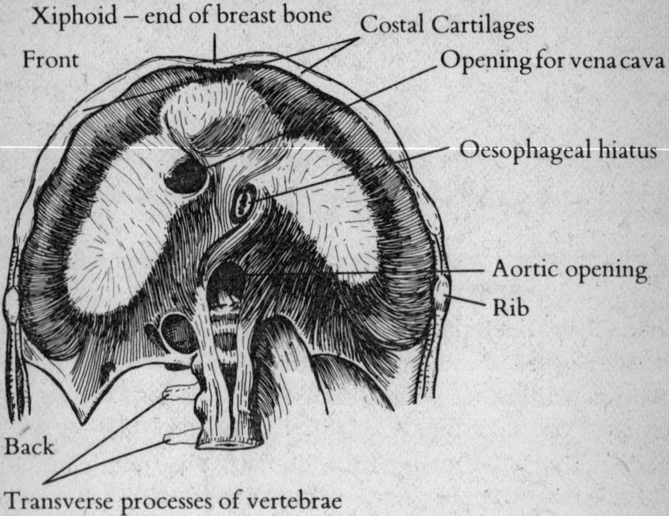

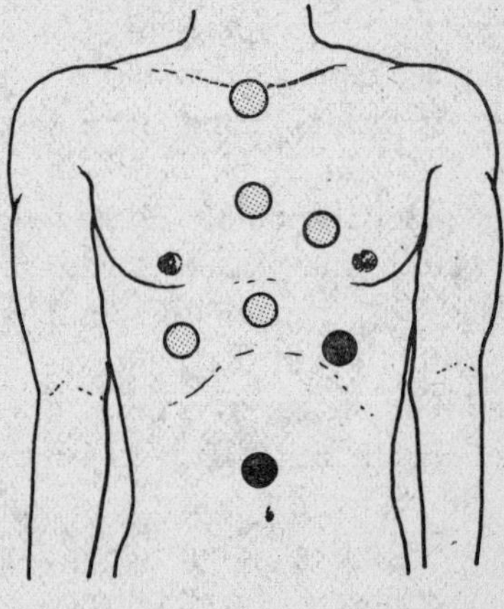

Different sites of pain

exact diagnosis, but a qualified diagnosis can be arrived at through the recognition of various symptoms. It is characterized by pain in several different areas. The commonest are behind the sternum (breast bone) at nipple level; and lower, behind the xiphoid process, at the end of the breast bone. Other areas of pain can be located on the left chest and may be mistaken for angina; at the base of the throat, or the right lower-ribs; and, more rarely, through the back behind the right shoulder blade.

Hiccups are sometimes symptomatic due to irritation of the phrenic nerve when the hernia is a large one. Pain increases on stooping with effort, and on lying down. 'Heart burn' is the usual description of the pain, and this is always worse after a meal. There is usually a feeling of fullness and bloatedness, and a considerable amount of flatulence is experienced. Intermittent nausea is cometimes complained of, and projectile vomiting can occur in severe cases.

2.
Causes of Hiatus Hernia

In naturopathic circles there is no doubt that the mechanical defect associated with hiatus hernia is caused by such twentieth-century western civilization factors as sedentary occupations, overweight, smoking and shallow breathing, impoverished diet, tight clothing and mental and emotional tension.

SEDENTARY OCCUPATIONS

Without sensible, that is regular, exercise, the system is predisposed to various types of ailments because cell activity is diminished. This means that elimination of waste matter is slowed and incomplete. Assimilation is also retarded and so metabolism is at a lower level. This results in toxic matter accumulating in the body, and in functional quality being reduced.

It is *not* a good idea to offset a sedentary job by violent exertion at weekends. Too much stress and strain is thrust upon a body which is unprepared and unfiit for strenuous activity. Steady, progressive training is the best plan, and if this is not possible, then gentler exercise, such as noncompetitive walking or swimming should be included in the weekly routine. Too much use of the car and lack of physical activity at work is responsible for many mechanical difficulties in the body, including spinal problems, varicose veins, constipation and so on, although these are also associated with an impoverished dietetic background.

OVERWEIGHT

This is due to overeating; either nibbling between meals, or eating too much at meal times, or a combination of both. The large meals are the greater danger in the condition we are discussing, because they increase the mechanical pressure on the diaphragm from the greatly distended stomach. However, overweight is always debilitating and taxing to the body, and it leads to diminished cell activity, reduced metabolism and a general 'below par' feeling. The adipose tissue also mechanically compresses the diaphragm and abdominal organs from without, inhibiting movement and proper organic function, often resulting in constipation which intensifies the toxic state.

SMOKING AND SHALLOW BREATHING

Smoking is a menace in any condition. It is already known how much lung cancer is caused by smoking. Not only this, but the *entire* level of health is lowered by the impoverished air circulating in the lungs and therefore in the bloodstream which, as a result, is unable to take oxygen to the tissues, or to absorb all the carbon dioxide from them. The absorption of vitamin B is inhibited and so the nervous system is made more vulnerable. This creates a vicious circle since smoking is erroneously thought to 'steady' the nerves. When lack of exercise coincides with the intake of stodgy, over refined and rich foods, it can be seen how the interconnected systems are put at considerable risk, and prevented from producing anything approaching well-being and wholeness.

Shallow breathing may be a result of smoking, or it may be caused by tight clothing, or by tension through daily pressures and anxiety. Shallow breathing occurs when the diaphragm is held tightly and only the upper chest moves during inhalation and exhalation. Therefore, due to lack of use, or little use, the muscle tone is diminished and so renders the diaphragm more liable to herniation. Added to this, shallow breathing inadequately aerates the lungs, and this results in less toxic elimination and less absorption of oxygen. Thorough interchange of gases in the lungs is essential to good health.

It can easily be understood, then, that smoking and shallow breathing predispose the 'victim' to many disorders: respiratory, digestive, circulatory and nervous.

IMPOVERISHED DIET

There are so many unwholesome products which come under the heading of 'food' today: for instance, all the cakes and biscuits and bread containing refined white flour; preservatives in meat, including sausages and delicatessen salamis; chemicals, improvers and flavourings added to ice-cream and squashes – not to mention refined sugar and syrups and an excess of salt in many packeted and easy-cook products such as instant mashed potato, custard powders and so on.

All these things should be avoided, since eating much devitalized and refined foods results in far less oxygen being introduced into the body than is required. Fewer mineral salts and vitamins are made available to balance and activate proper nutrition, and in addition there is too little fibre present to stimulate the peristaltic action of the colon and keep it healthy. As a result, all body tissues function at less than their full potential, indeed, less than their average potential. Muscle tone is weakened, and the muscles become less resilient, and connective and fibrous tissue suffers through pour nourishment, and is consequently more prone to decomposition and damage. Also the mucous membranes become thinned and more easily irritated.

Drinks, too, can be harmful. Tea and coffee both irritate the nervous system and the digestive tract, and leave acid wastes that slow down elimination. Squashes, coffee, and alcohol all affect the mucous lining of the stomach. When these drinks are taken with meals or immediately afterwards the weight of the stomach content is increased, stretching the stomach wall. This unwise mixture also encourages fermentation and produces gas; thus the distension of the stomach is increased, causing pressure against the diaphragm and the oesophageal opening, and greatly increasing the risk of herniation.

'We are what we eat', so it is up to every individual to eat a fully balanced diet which provides the body with all the necessary raw materials for its proper function. In this way health is maintained and disease prevented. A healthy regime should consist of *at least* fifty per cent fruit and vegetables, and half of that amount should be uncooked. The other food categories, carbohydrates, proteins and fats should make up the other fifty per cent. When we really do eat and drink wisely, the functional standard of all the body systems improves. As a result we think more clearly and act with greater precision and awareness.

TIGHT CLOTHING

Restriction of movement around the waist causes compression. This reacts on the digestive, nervous and circulatory systems, but particularly on the diaphragm and respiratory system. Movement is restricted, and the body functions are undermined. Many women choose to wear a bra and girdle which overlap at the waist to control a 'spare tyre'. Though this may achieve its objective, such clothing is really detrimental to health, and is a strong predisposing factor in the condition of hiatus hernia.

MENTAL AND EMOTIONAL TENSION

All emotional and mental tensions and upsets react on the vagus nerve and sympathetic nervous system. The most easily recognized area affected is the solar plexus – where the feeling of 'butterflies' occurs when we are anxious. In such instances the solar plexus tightens up and the feeling experienced is like a hard lump. We all know the horrible, sick feeling experienced when we pass an accident on the road. Jealousy, anger, resentment and self-pity all react on this finely tuned 'relay station' whose function is to get adrenalin flowing and to increase the heart beat and rate of blood flow. Further metabolic changes include faster breathing to correspond with an increased pulse rate; a retarding of the digestive functions and the repair and growth processes. When chronic anxiety occurs all this takes place, though less noticeably, diminishing function and inhibiting diaphragmatic movement, which is so essential to good health and the prevention of hiatus hernia.

3.
The Holistic Treatment of Hiatus Hernia

What can be done? It is obviously necessary to rehabilitate the whole body; a momentous task indeed, but taken slowly, step by step, with a positive persistence, the new regime will not be too difficult and, as the body systems are relieved, encouragement is found to persevere. Before beginning the actual treatment, it is advisable to raise the head end of the bed, either by using bricks to stand the legs of the bed on, or by wedging the mattress higher, using a very firm bolster, a piece of wood or wedge-shaped foam rubber. This helps to prevent the regurgitation of food during the night. More pillows can also be used.

RELAXATION

It is first important to learn to breathe properly; that is, using the diaphragm and, by doing this, beginning to learn to relax. Diaphragmatic breathing is quite easy really, and the following routine is to be recommended.

Lie down with both knees bent and feet close to buttocks; feel relaxed, put both hands lightly on the abdomen and concentrate the attention on this area. Now breathe in, gently pushing the abdomen up under the hands at the same time, until no more air can be inhaled. Then relax, breathing out through the mouth with an audible sighing sound and allowing the abdominal wall to sink back (see diagram). The shoulders and chest should remain at rest throughout.

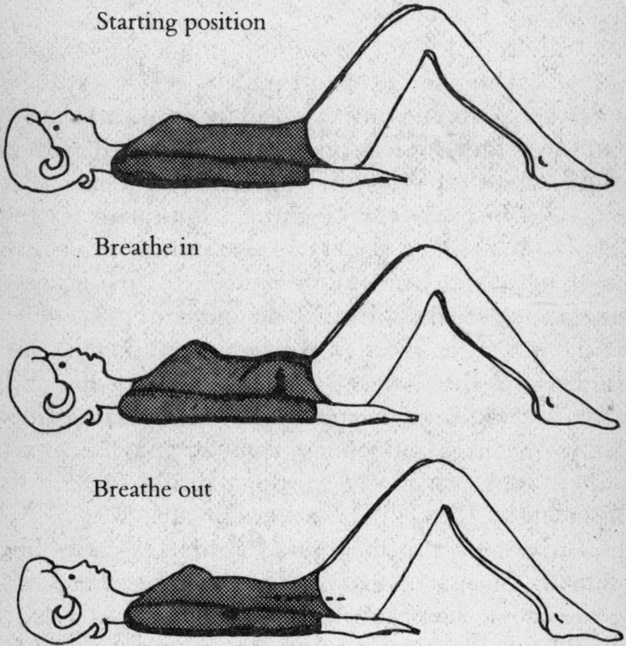

Diaphragmatic breathing

At first, there might be a desire to 'suck in' the abdomen and expand the chest, because this is what is understood by 'deep breathing', and some methods of teaching emphasize chest expansion as the most important part of respiration. It certainly does play a part, but the use of the diaphragm increases the capacity of the lungs from above, downwards. Rhythmical movement, or athletic training to increase lung capacity exerts a massaging effect on the abdominal organs, stimulating good function.

A really complete breath begins with the diaphragm and continues with the intercostal muscles which expand the lungs from above, downwards, and from side to side. Try a complete breath once or twice. It would be exhausting to breathe in such a way for long, but it is very useful in exercising. In every day conditions, breathing is a reflex action and, unless the diaphragm is influenced in a negative way – by anxiety, tension or holding the tummy in for appearance sake, it performs its function well.

Back then to the practice. It is best done first thing in the morning and last thing at night. Begin with five or six 'tummy' breaths, increasing by one each day to fifteen. Always be at ease – no forcing. If any strain is felt, then too much effort is being used; working hard at it defeats the purpose. Get up slowly afterwards (at the morning session), as deep breathing usually causes a slight feeling of giddiness. This is normal, and is due to acceleration of the circulation and passes off after a few seconds. During the day, just occasionally, try to do the same type of breathing while sitting, well supported, in a chair; then, while standing and walking. However, don't worry if it doesn't seem to work. The very action of directing thought to the diaphragm helps to promote its function, and the exercise will get easier each time. This type of breathing will relieve pain, so it should be practised whenever there is an attack.

It is important to be able to relax at any time and, through the learning and application of this skill, to prevent bodily and mental tensions from building up into proportions that cause actual physical symptoms. To begin then, lie down on a hard surface, (though it may be uncomfortable to start with, it is more difficult to cheat yourself and has more teaching value than a soft bed or couch); the floor, with a sleeping bag to make it a little more acceptable and warmer is good or, in fine summer weather, the garden lawn would be splendid, with a rug – relaxation is impossible in cold conditions.

Part of learning to relax is to try to be aware of the body in a positive way. With real awareness comes the ability to recognize stress-tension at once, and the build-up cannot occur if it (the stress) is released in the first instance. To make the contrast between tension and relaxation more vivid to the learner, a series of deliberate actions of tensing and releasing several different muscle and joint groups is practised, beginning with the feet and working up to the head. It is done in harmony with the breathing, in this manner:

1. Breathe in, and bend the feet up to ninety degrees. Hold for a few seconds, noting the tautness in the shin muscles and ankle joints. Breathe out to a sigh and 'let go' – don't try to *do* anything in this half of the movement, simply release the tension caused by bending the feet up. Repeat once.

2. Move your attention up to the knees. Breathe in as you press both knees on to the ground, noting the tautness in the thigh muscles. Breathe out to a sigh and release them. Repeat.
3. Move your attention to the buttocks. Breathe in and contract (squeeze) these big muscles together. (Try not to tighten any other area of the body. You may catch yourself clenching hands or jaws to 'assist', but this must be prevented). Note the tension as before, and then release it while breathing out and sighing. Repeat.
4. Think about your abdominal area (tummy). Draw these muscles back, as if to touch your spine while breathing in (the reverse of diaphragmatic breathing). Hold for a few seconds, noticing the discomfort, and then breathe out and release the muscles. Repeat.
5. The hands are next on the list – clench them both really tightly increasing the grip as you breathe in – you can really feel the 'blocking' that tension will cause. Breathe out sighing and release the hands. It should give quite a sense of relief if the clenching was strong. Repeat.
6. Bend the elbows hard, hands up to shoulders, breathing in – breathe out and release as before. Repeat.
7. Next, while breathing in, draw the shoulder blades together tightly, note the discomfort, and release it while sighing. Repeat.
8. Now the face muscles – screw up the muscles around the eyes, frown, clench the jaw, all while breathing in. Then release it with a sigh. Repeat.

   Finish off this preliminary section by adding all the 'tensings' together and stiffen the whole body, then 'fall in a heap', so to speak, while releasing and sighing out. Repeat.

It takes quite an effort to do this, and the relief of letting go is very noticeable. Follow this with three or four slow, deep diaphragmatic breaths, still sighing as you breathe out. Begin to still your mind by deliberately remembering a beautiful place – somewhere special to you – quiet and deserted, and, in imagination, put yourself there. Explore it in your mind's eye and appreciate its beauty deeply; feel yourself as part of this beauty. Ignore your body, and expand into these lovely surroundings. Imagine yourself to be part of the universe, (which you are), essential in the scheme of things. Feel contented, at peace, warm and drowsy and just stay there for a few minutes (or as long as you can). Presently, leave the lovely place, come back to the present, yawn and stretch and 'wake up'. Get up gradually because resting slows down metabolism and to hurry up might involve a slight shock to the system.

Incidentally, if you are within hearing of a telephone, either bury it in cushions or take it off the hook. As you can understand, the aim of all this is to become completely detached from everyday things for a while and allow mind and body to rest and recharge. Practised every day, taking say ten, then twenty minutes, working up to half an hour, your conscious mind, and also the subconscious will be trained and, in time, you will realize that you are not getting so 'up tight' about things, that worry doesn't penetrate so deeply and that you are calmer. This regime is tremendously helpful in any condition where anxiety and tension is a factor.

DIETETIC MEANS

Now we come to the point where preconceived ideas have to be unlearnt and new thoughts adopted; so that it is necessary to be willing to adapt to a fresh outlook and to try out the new approach with an open mind.

Begin by giving up smoking or, if preferred, cut down by two cigarettes a day, steadily. Although this will prove difficult, keep in mind the fact that the whole body is going to benefit once the withdrawal problems are over. Allow one cup (not mug) of decaffeinated coffee and one cup of tea each day. At other times, have fruit or vegetable juices, herbal teas or beverages such as 'barley cup' or a dandelion coffee. There is a wide choice, all obtainable at health food shops. At the same time, remember to observe separate eating and drinking times; take fluids half an hour before a meal, or two hours afterwards. This helps the digestive process considerably and reduces the incidence of 'heart burn'. Drinking with meals increases the over-all weight in the stomach, slows down the digestive process by diluting the digestive juices and this increases the risk of fermentation and gas formation, which distends the stomach and causes pressure again, and therefore, discomfort and pain.

All meals should be smaller in quantity than usual, and thorough mastication is essential, both to break up the food into really small particles, and to slow down the rate of intake. A rough estimate would be about thirty-two to forty chews for each mouthful. Please do *not* count every mouthful eaten. Be conscious of chewing more thoroughly and, now and then, count, just to see how near the mark you get. Obviously, it will depend on the type of food eaten, and this introduces another point; on the whole, the diet will consist of more fruit and vegetables than before and less soft, refined, and over-processed things like white bread and sugar, cakes and biscuits, rice puddings and overcooked vegetables. It was mentioned at the beginning, and repetition will help to emphasize, that diets in general should consist of at least fifty per cent fruit and vegetables, and fifty per cent, collectively, of protein, carbohydrates and fat.

In the case of the hiatus hernia, it is very important to introduce raw juices into the diet as soon as possible. However, the digestive tract will probably be hypersensitive at first; therefore, it is suggested that raw, freshly made carrot juice be sipped half an hour before each meal. Yes, even before breakfast. In the absence of a juicing gadget it can still be prepared quite simply, and instructions follow, together with sample menus and recipes later in the booklet. Carrot juice has a very restorative effect, as it is rich in vitamin A and calcium, and is also an alkaline substance, which soothes the stomach. Persevere with this, though admittedly, carrot juice tastes rather insipid. Note here that all juices, whether fruit or vegetable, should be slightly diluted because they are concentrated. Always add one tablespoon of water to them; either tap or bottled water should, very definitely, be used. Variations can be made later, by mixing fresh apple juice with the carrot, and by using beetroot and apple juice together, or beetroot and celery – (these latter really need a proper juicer). The bottled varieties are quite good, but they have had to be pasteurized, so some vitamin and oxygen content is lost. Nevertheless, it is a convenient and less messy way of obtaining juices.

It is worth metnioning that beetroots, in any quantity, cause colouration of the urine (pink) and faeces (dark red). This is normal, and not a symptom of disease.

It is a good plan to begin the day well by introducing something beneficial into the body. So instead of the usual cup of tea, which over-stimulates the nervous system, irritates the lining of the stomach, and increases acidity in the blood stream, have a herbal tea. These have a gentler effect and activate the healing resources of the body, so that a better balance is possible. *Mint* tea aids digestion, disperses flatulence and tones up the lining of the stomach. *Chamomile* soothes the nervous system and is good for colic; so either is excellent first thing in the morning and, taken alternately, you get the best of both.

Always allow hot drinks to cool a little before taking. Extremes of temperature, in both food and drink, should be avoided; and just as food should be eaten slowly, so should drinks be sipped.

Some readers may find it better suited to their particular temperament and the regime of the home to make the changes really slowly. Natural processes are slow, and it is far better to make changes slowly and consistently, than to rush into a situation and then be unable to maintain it. In addition, too many sudden changes can cause a reaction in the body, perhaps temporarily increasing symptoms which could act as a deterrent to further dieting.

Week One

Use this week as follows:

1. Learn the breathing and relaxation.
2. Drink 4 fl oz of freshly made carrot juice before each meal. Remember, this should be SIPPED.
3. Drink and eat at separate times.

4. If necessary, cut out (or down) smoking.
5. Drink only one cup of tea and one cup of decaffeinated coffee (or a substitute) per day.
6. Begin the day with mint or chamomile tea.
7. Eat smaller meals, and chew them very well.
8. Raise the bed-head level by six inches and generally get into the feel of the new regime. Prepare to let the natural forces in the body take over and redress the imbalance that has been going on for so long and, in time, all the above eight factors cannot fail to produce improvement; indeed, any one of them would help a little.

The second week will require following a stricter plan, aimed at cleansing the body of toxic wastes and stimulating repair processes, at the same time relieving pain and discomfort.

The diet will be very simple at first, using natural whole foods and few mixtures, as an aid to digestion. Gradually, more foods, rich in oxygen, vitamins and minerals will be introduced, to promote healing and health. A full diet, based on whole foods of course, and preferably vegetarian will then be suggested at the end of the course. This phase, the last one concerning the hiatus hernia, will be the first phase of a new way of life, with no going back to the old, unhealthy habits. It should be a life of increased vitality, and greater capacity, both for work and enjoyment; a life of broader concepts and spiritual awareness; a life of sound health.

Week Two

The basic food for the week is brown rice because it contains silica, a mineral which helps the body to throw off (eliminate) toxic matter and also helps to initiate healing, especially in digestive problems. Brown rice still retains its natural bran, which is more delicate than wheat bran, and so provides bulk for the system, without irritation. Rice is largely a starch food, but it has about eight per cent protein content, as well as traces of calcium and phosphorous and, more importantly, several of the B vitamins – thiamine, niacin and, to a lesser extent, riboflavin. These vitamins are valuable in nourishing the nervous system, as is well known.

The three main meals will be rice-based. The grain is boiled, and it would save a lot of effort if a quantity were cooked to last for two days. Wash half a pound of rice in a sieve, and drop it into one pint of boiling water, to which one teaspoon of sunflower oil has been added. (This helps to keep the grains separate). Allow to boil slowly, until all the moisture has been absorbed – about twenty to twenty-five minutes. Turn out into a basin or container with a lid, and it is ready; keep in the fridge or a cool place. The amount recommended will be small, deliberately so, but if you are really needing more, a little extra may be added.

Day One

7 a.m.	On waking, mint or chamomile tea.
8 a.m.	4 fl oz freshly made carrot juice.
8.30 a.m.	Breakfast: 3 level tablespoonsful of boiled rice; 3 tablespoonsful of stewed apple (sweetened with honey).
10.30 a.m.	Barley cup (this may be warmed up if preferred).
12.30 p.m.	Carrot juice.

1 p.m. Lunch: 3 tablespoonsful of rice with one tablespoonful of finely grated raw carrot and one tablespoonful of finely chopped parsley. (This provides vitamins A and C, calcium and potassium.) A very little yeast extract savoury or soy sauce can be added.

3 p.m. China tea or herb tea.

5 p.m. Carrot juice.

5.30 p.m. Evening meal: 3 tablespoonsful of rice with 4 to 6 prunes or apricots that have been soaked overnight, not cooked, and 2 tablespoonsful of natural yogurt.

7.30 p.m. Barley cup or herb tea, followed at bedtime by 4fl oz red grape juice with a generous splash of mineral water. This is a good sedative drink and a digestive as well.

Sleep should be good when following this plan, as there will be no food in the stomach by bedtime; and by having the night drink half an hour before going to bed, that too will be well on its way through the digestive tract. Diaphragmatic breathing will also help induce sleep.

Day Two

This is a repetition of the first day, though amounts may need to be varied a little. It is important that the lower bowel be kept free; and as the total amount of bulk being taken in is less than usual, there may be temporary difficulty. If this second day passes without any action, then there is the choice between taking a herbal laxative and using a small, warm water enema – about one and a half pints would be enough. This treatment will depend on whether there is someone to administer it – or it could be self-administered if the patient is confident about it.

Day Three

This is a progressive diet and the aim, throughout, is to increase the amount of raw foods taken, as these encourage healing and raise the level of health generally. When accompanied by whole cereals, vegetable and grain protein, unsaturated oils and natural sugars, a real balance is achieved. Individuals differ, of course, and, in offering general advice, it is impossible to cater for special needs. To the reader who feels the need of personal support, please consult a qualified naturopath.

7 a.m.	Herbal tea as before.
8 a.m.	Fresh carrot juice.
8.30 a.m.	Breakfast: 3 to 4 tablespoonsful of boiled rice with 6 prunes or apricots, 2 tablespoonsful natural yogurt and a tablespoonful of ground almonds.
10.30 a.m.	Barley cup or similar.
12.30 p.m.	Fresh carrot juice.
1 p.m.	Lunch: 3 to 4 tablespoonsful of boiled brown rice with 1 tablespoonsful of grated raw carrot, a teaspoonful of chopped parsley, a teaspoonful of sunflower seeds, 6 to 8 sprigs of watercress, chopped and mixed into the rice with 1 or 2 tablespoonsful of natural yogurt and a small amount, say half a teaspoonful, of some yeast extract savoury.

3.30 p.m. China tea or herbal tea.
5.30 p.m. Carrot juice.
6.00 p.m. Evening meal: Brown rice, as before, mixed with one grated raw apple including skin and pips, soaked prunes or apricots, a tablespoonful of ground almonds and 2 tablespoonsful of natural yogurt (with a little honey if necessary).
8.30 p.m. Barley cup or mint tea.
9.30/
10 p.m. Red grape juice as before.

Day Four

This is a repetition of Day Three. By now, considering this is the second week, a definite lessening of symptoms will be experienced and a little more energy will be available. Certainly, the nervous system will be calmer. Each day, the diet will get more interesting.

Day Five

The routine as before, with the waking drink and carrot juice.

Breakfast: A grated raw apple, 4 to 6 prunes or apricots, a tablespoonful of ground almonds, 2 tablespoonsful of natural yogurt and a ripe banana.
Mid-morning: Barley cup or dandelion coffee or apple juice.
Before lunch: Tomato juice.
Lunch: 4 oz cottage cheese, into which mix a teaspoonful of chopped mint, a grated carrot, a teaspoonful of sunflower seeds, a dessertspoonful of raisins, a tomato (scalded and the

skin removed), a teaspoonful of cider vinegar and a few sprigs of watercress.

Mid-afternoon: Herbal or China tea or bottled fruit juice (apple or pineapple).

Before the evening meal: Carrot or tomato juice.

Evening meal: 2 potatoes (small), steamed with their skins on, 2 carrots (small), 2 oz of frozen peas, a teaspoonful of polyunsaturated margarine and a teaspoonful of yeast extract.

Routine as before to finish the evening.

Day Six

Repeat Day Five.

Day Seven

Maintain the usual routine for between meals.

Breakfast: 'Muesli': Overnight soak 2 tablespoonsful of flaked oats or wheat in 4 tablespoonsful of cold water. In the morning, add: a grated raw apple, a dessertspoonful of raisins, 8 chopped almonds, a dessertspoonful of powdered milk (or 2 tablespoonsful of yogurt) and a teaspoonful of honey. Chew this really well.

Lunch: 2 or 3 lettuce leaves, 4 or 5 sprigs of watercress, a skinned tomato, a grated raw carrot, a small grated raw beetroot, sunflower seeds, half an apple, chopped or grated, 4 oz cottage cheese, 2 teaspoonsful cider vinegar sprinkled over 1 or 2 steamed potatoes with skin still on.

Evening meal: Steamed vegetables: $\frac{1}{4}$ heart of cabbage (if not too big), 2 carrots, a small onion, $\frac{1}{2}$ a red or green pepper, sliced into the cabbage and steamed together. 2 oz grated

Cheshire cheese to sprinkle over. (*Note:* Peppers are a rich source of vitamin C and retain quite an amount of it even when cooked.)

This completes the second week. Now make an assessment – weigh yourself. How successful have you been in your estimation? Are you pleased with your progress? Do you still feel hungry after meals? If so, this will pass as your stomach returns to normal size. As the meals become slightly more comprehensive, do you still suffer pain or flatulence? The flatulence may persist for weeks yet, but should be less severe in frequency and volume. Do you feel more relaxed and optimistic? Make a list of what yet needs to be achieved, and feel pleased and confident with your progress so far.

Week Three

Quite a number of changes will be made in the diet this week, progressing to a full normal reformed diet in the fourth week. These changes may be too rapid for some, and slight regression might occur. If this is the case, return to the stage that provided most comfort for a few more days and then try the progression again. There is no merit in forcing on if it has a negative effect.

Day One

First thing: On waking, 2 teaspoonsful of cider vinegar and a little honey in hot water.
Before breakfast: 4 fl oz of bottled apple juice.
Breakfast: 'Muesli' with prunes and yogurt.
11 a.m. Coffee-type drink.
Before lunch: Vegetable juice: choose from carrot, beetroot,

celery, tomato, or a mixture of any two. Take 4 fl oz as usual.

Lunch: Salad: Keep amounts small. Use a sliced pepper, lettuce, watercress, beetroot, carrot, sunflower seeds, tomato, cottage cheese and mint. For the starch requirement have 100 per cent wholewheat bread and polyunsaturated margarine. Just eat one slice at present. For dessert, an apple.

4 p.m. China or herb tea, as before.

Before the evening meal: Grapefruit juice.

Evening meal: Poached egg on mashed carrots with green vegetable in season, and a potato in skin. For dessert, an apple or pear.

2 hours later: A coffee type drink if needed.

Before bed: The usual grape juice.

Day Two

First thing: On waking, cider vinegar as before.

Before breakfast: Apple juice as before.

Breakfast: A banana, 8 almonds, 8 dates, an apple, yogurt or 4 fl oz untreated milk.

11 a.m. Grapefruit juice.

Before lunch: Mineral water.

Lunch: Salad mixture as before, but have 2 oz milled nuts (not peanuts) as protein, and potato as starch. For dessert, an apple.

4 p.m. Tea as before.

Before the evening meal: Grapefruit juice.

Evening meal: Grilled white fish – haddock, cod or plaice fillet, with carrots and peas. For dessert, grapes or pear. Follow this with the usual bedtime drink.

Day Three
First thing: Early drinks as before.
Breakfast: A boiled egg, a slice of 100 per cent wholemeal bread with polyunsaturated margarine. One or two apples.
Mid-morning: Grapefruit juice.
Before lunch: Mineral water.
Lunch: Salad: Try different ingredients, e.g. celery or cucumber, 2 oz Cheddar cheese, and 1 or 2 potatoes. For dessert, soaked prunes and/or apricots.
4 p.m. Tea as usual.
Before evening meal: Pineapple juice.
Evening meal: Millet and Tomato Savoury* with carrots, and green vegetables. For dessert, grapes or a pear.

To complete the week repeat the three days already given, and then Day One again. If the diet has been adhered to and progress has been made the fourth week can be started with confidence.

Week Four
Monday
First thing: Choose between cider vinegar, fruit juices and herb tea.
Before breakfast: Mineral water.
Breakfast: Fruit and natural yogurt with a little honey, an apple, 8 to 12 grapes and a pear. The yogurt can be eaten straight or the whole thing made into a fruit salad and the yogurt poured over.
Mid-morning: Savoury yeast extract drink diluted with milk

* See recipe section.

and water, carrot juice or herb tea.
Before lunch: Pineapple juice.
Lunch: Salad: Lettuce, tomato (skinned), grated carrot and beetroot, sliced pepper (a little), sprouted alfalfa seeds (see page 59), two small slices of 100 per cent wholewheat bread and unsalted butter. A hard-boiled egg. Use cider vinegar and sunflower oil as salad dressing, or alternatively yogurt. Fresh fruit as dessert.
Mid-afternoon: China tea.
Before the evening meal: Pineapple juice.
Evening meal: First course: Half an avocado with vinaigrette dressing.
Second course: Cauliflower, carrots, courgettes (in season), 2 oz grated Cheddar cheese to sprinkle over the vegetables. Fresh fruit to follow.
Evening drinks as before.

Tuesday
Note: Before and between breakfast, lunch, and the evening meal, drinks should follow the same pattern as before.
Breakfast: Soaked prunes and apricots, a teaspoonful of sunflower seeds, a dessertspoonful of ground almonds, natural yogurt.
Lunch: Salad: Watercress and orange, celery, beetroot. Dressing: Yogurt and chopped mint. Try potato and cottage cheese with this. Eat as much as you feel comfortable with.
Fresh fruit to follow.
Evening meal: First course: Avocado with vinaigrette dressing

Second course: Mushroom omelette, peas or runner beans, and carrots.
Dessert: Apple Crumble*.

Wednesday
(Keep to the drinking pattern)
Breakfast: A boiled egg, two slices of 100 per cent wholemeal bread and polyunsaturated margarine, and an apple.
Lunch: Grated carrot, grated apple, grated raw beetroot, a tablespoonful of sunflower seeds, a teaspoonful of chopped parsley, 4 oz of cottage cheese, two rye crispbreads and polyunsaturated margarine. French dressing.
A *ripe* banana and yogurt to follow.
Evening meal: First course: Half a grapefruit.
Second course: Soya Savoury*, green vegetables (e.g. cabbage), carrots, leeks (in season) or onions.
Dessert: Soaked prunes and apricots with goat's milk yogurt.

Thursday
Breakfast: Home-made Muesli*.
Lunch: Mixed salad: Lettuce, watercress, tomato (skinned), raw grated courgette (a small one), grated carrot, a few raisins, a slice of onion, yogurt and mint dressing. A slice of 100 per cent wholewheat bread and butter, and a tablespoonful of ground almonds.
Evening meal: First course: Tomato salad.
Second course: Egg and Cheese Savoury,* with peas or runner beans, carrots and courgettes.
Dessert: Fresh fruit.

* See recipe section.

Friday
Breakfast: Fresh fruit: Grapes, an orange, an apple and a few dates and nuts, preferably almonds or hazelnuts.
Lunch: Salad: Sprouted alfalfa seeds, coleslaw or raw cabbage, carrots with a little onion, and vinaigrette dressing. One or two potatoes, Soaked prunes or apricots to follow.
Evening meal: First course: Half a grapefruit.
Second course: Stuffed pepper, carrots and green vegetables (in season).
Dessert: Baked apples, stuffed with raisins or dates.

Saturday
Breakfast: A sliced ripe banana, raisins, sunflower seeds and natural yogurt.
Lunch: Salad: Mixed cooked beetroot and celery, apple and walnut tossed in vinaigrette dressing, two rye crispbreads with cottage cheese.
Fresh fruit – grapes or peaches (in season).
Evening meal: First course: Tomato salad.
Second course: Chestnut Pudding,* with green vegetables, carrots and peas.
Dessert: Fresh fruit salad.

Sunday
Breakfast: Scrambled eggs on toast and an apple.
Lunch: First course: Half a grapefruit.
Second course: Cauliflower cheese, courgettes and carrots.
Dessert: Baked apples.
Evening meal: Fresh fruit: An apple, an orange, grapes, nuts and raisins.

* See recipe section.

These four weeks should have given you an understanding of how to continue dietetically. Apart from a possible increase in quantities, the overall pattern should remain similar. Care must be taken not to increase the quantities too much because of the risk that an over-full stomach may protrude through the oesophageal opening. By avoiding such pressure, and by eating wholesome nourishing foods, the chances of the hernia actually healing are greatly increased.

EXERCISE

It was said in an earlier section that exercise not only keeps muscles in good tone, but affects the tissues throughout the body by rhythmical cell activity. Short bursts of exercise are really not helpful; and just to run through a few exercises for ten minutes daily only helps to keep the body flexible, (though this is good), without having any deeper effect on cell activity. It is this deeper effect that is necessary for treating hiatus hernia, as well as for improving the abdominal muscle tone.

A good walk is excellent for this purpose. It should last at least thirty to forty minutes, building up to an hour, if possible. At the beginning, it may be necessary for some individuals to be more cautious. It would be a mistake to take on a long walk if quite unprepared for it. A regular walk say for twenty minutes, is not without value, and the length can be gradually increased. This would be preferable to taking on the longer walk and getting overtired, and being put off from doing any more. If carried out in this way, walking produces a mild glow or sweat, which shows that the whole system is activated, and elimination is accelerated through the lungs and skin, leaving less toxic matter to clog the body.

Getting rid of waste matter is always important to health, and it is because many people are unaware of this principle in its entirety, only being taught to watch bowel action and thereby neglecting the lungs and skin, that overloading so often occurs. Frequently, too, bowel action is less than adequate, unfortunately. However, if a good diet and regular exercise are observed, all these inequalities rebalance themselves through the innate intelligence of body cells, which are health-orientated.

Our bodies, then, are always working towards *health*. If we only learnt not to throw spanners in the works by bad diet and bad habits generally, the level of good health experienced would be incredibly higher.

There are several specific exercises for the abdominal muscles, and these will be beneficial if practised regularly and rhythmically. It would probably be advisable to graduate the time factor for those who are weak or unfamiliar with exercising, but generally fifteen to twenty minutes daily would be the average time necessary for maximum effect. (The most important exercise – deep diaphragmatic breathing – has already been described.)

The practice of these exercises, for ten minutes to begin with, increasing to twenty, will help specifically, but also will increase body awareness, and thereby improve posture. All too frequently, because of rushing, tiredness, and the effect of gravity, we all tend to sink and slump down, nevertheless remaining tense at the same time. It is really important that we become aware of this and lift ourselves up, as such exercise has both a physical and psychological effect, and is of great benefit. However, do not go to the other extreme and become rigid in the stretched up position! No, just lift the rib cage lightly, lowering and relaxing the shoulders, and stretching the back of the neck and top of the head easily. Immediately, this produces a feeling of greater control and integration and ability to cope with the daily round. So next time you feel 'down in the dumps', lift yourself up, remembering the slow deep breathing. The same type of exercise is effective if you feel jittery and 'up tight'.

It is surprising how much can be done, both to prevent illness and to promote good health. Health awareness presents an exciting challenge, and a basis for continual learning and personal development.

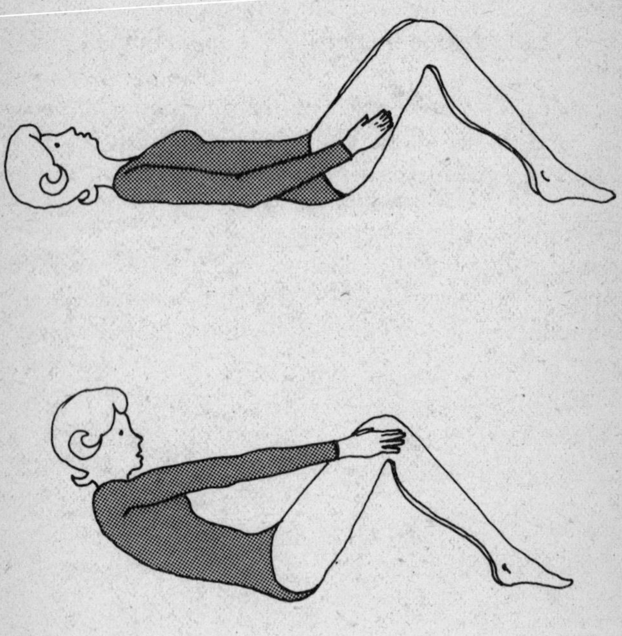

Lying in 'crook' position. Exercise 1

Exercise 1

Lie in a crook position – that is, with both knees bent and feet close to buttocks and arms at the sides. Place hands on thighs where they join the abdomen, and then slide them up to reach the knees, lifting the head and shoulders, and breathing in slowly. Breathe out while falling back and relaxing. Repeat four to six times. Notice how the abdominal muscles shorten as you reach forward.

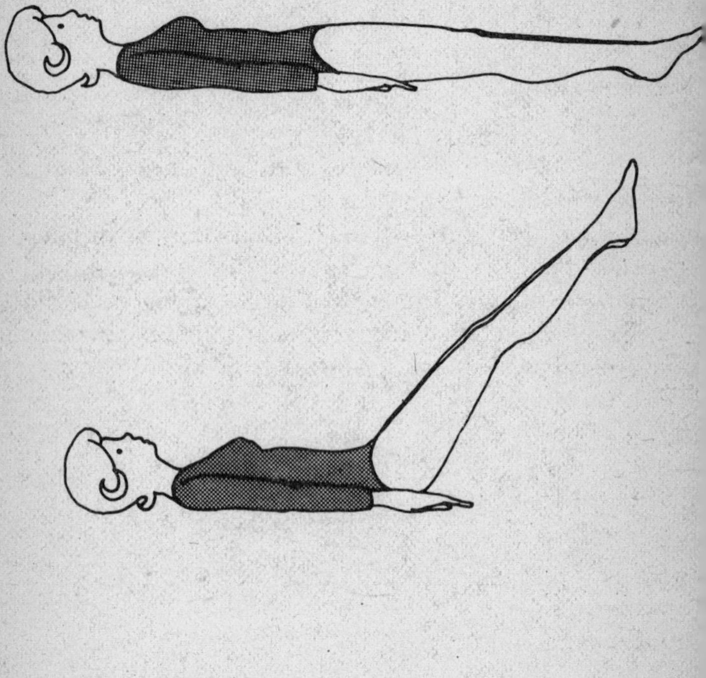

Exercise 2

Exercise 2

Lie flat on your back with legs out straight. Lift both legs together to 45°, breathing in slowly, then lower them, breathing out and relaxing. Repeat four times.

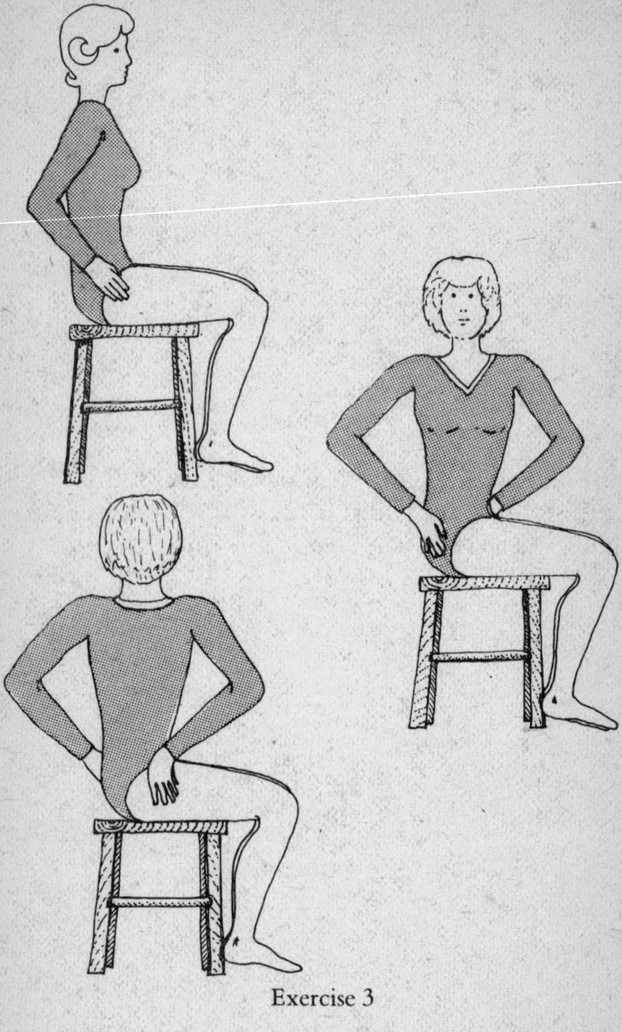

Exercise 3

Exercise 3

Sit on a stool, hands on hips. Use arms as levers, twisting round first to the right and then to the left. This movement takes place at the waist level. Look over each shoulder as you twist. Counting a right and left twist as one, repeat seven to ten times. No special breathing, but note that you do *not* have to hold your breath.

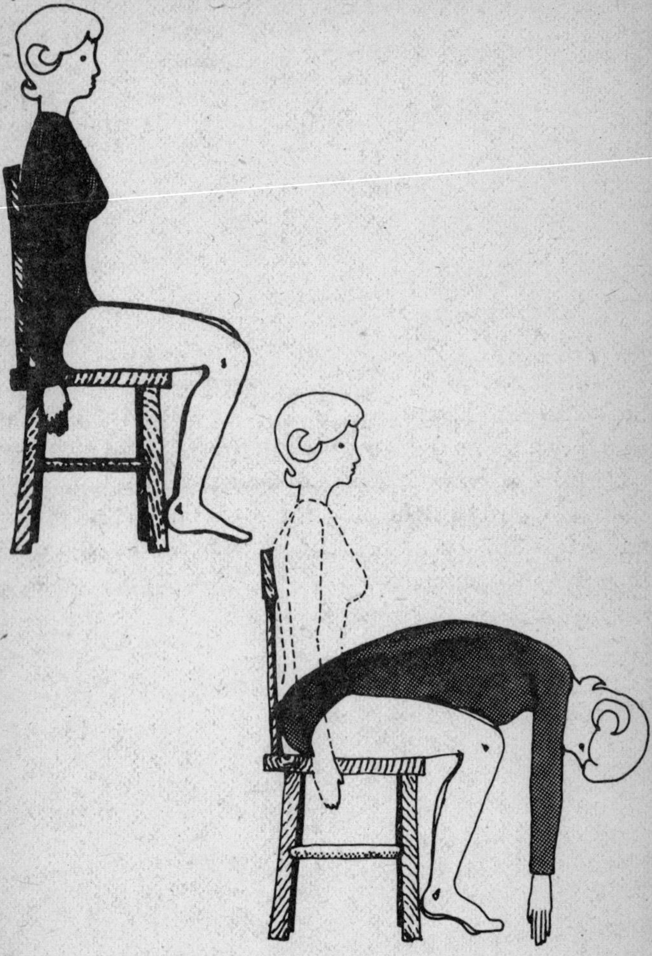

Exercise 4

Exercise 4
Sit on a straight-backed chair (kitchen type) with back supported and bottom tucked well back – arms at the sides. Relax forward, *breathing out* (head to knees). Uncurl, inching your back up against the back of the chair until upright *breathing in* slowly all the time. Remember to keep the head low until upright position is reached, and the back should be rounded and uncurling – not coming up in a stiff straight line. Repeat four times.

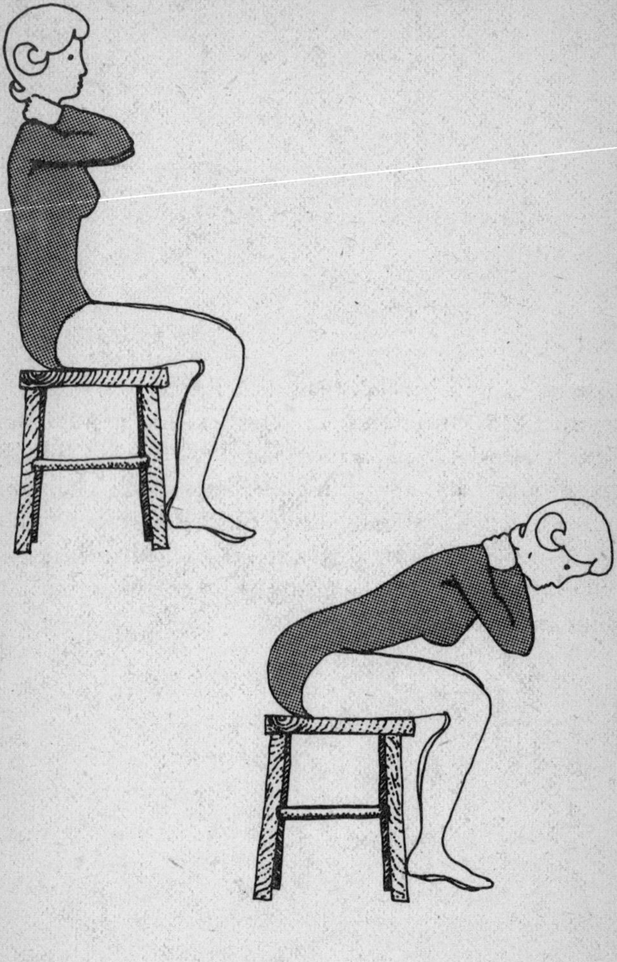

Exercise 5

Exercise 5
This one is designed to lift the rib cage and expand the chest. Sit as in *Exercise 4*. Clasp hands behind the neck, then drop head, shoulders and elbows forwards, breathing out. Raise head and brace elbows back – holding the chin in. Breathe in whilst raising up and expanding. Repeat five times.

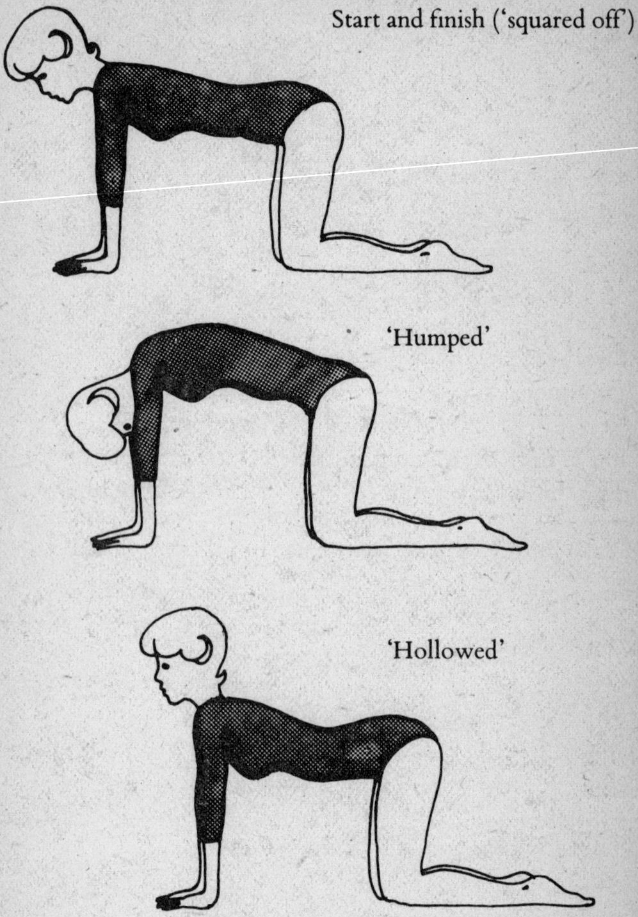

Exercise 6

Exercise 6

This one is designed for spine and chest mobility. Kneel in a 'donkey' position – on all fours, arms and thighs at right angles to body, spine straight. Bend head down; at the same time 'hump' the spine (all is rounded) and breathe in. Now change by 'hollowing' the lower back and raising the head back. Breathe out as you do so. Keep elbows rigid as arms and thighs act as pillars of support. Repeat six times.

HYDROTHERAPY

Water is another source of natural healing, and is usually undervalued. Cold water can have a tonic effect on blood vessels and nerves, especially in the skin. Hot water relaxes the body, but needs to be used with discretion. Hot and cold water, used in contrast, is very stimulating and beneficial in speeding up elimination, absorption and healing. Ice is useful in treating recent injuries, and prevents the body overreacting to damage. Cold compresses to localized areas provide a natural warmth, which relaxes and promotes absorption and elimination of toxic matter. Thus, self-provided warmth is preferable to heat which is applied from outside the body. Water can be very useful in regulating body temperature by the application of complete body packs to promote sweating, or by repeated sponging to bring down a high temperature.

Water has been used as a therapy from ancient times – the Greeks and Romans both realized its value, externally and internally. They developed a form of colonic lavage, employing an animals horn to convey the water into the rectum. So enemas and colonic wash-outs are nothing new!

In addition, there are or were the spa towns, centres where people went to 'take the water' – to drink it, or bathe in it or both. Unfortunately, most of the English centres have closed – Cheltenham, Bath, Buxton – but those on the continent seem to have been maintained.

The use of water in the case of hiatus hernia, takes the form of cold packs applied to the upper abdominal area. The rationale behind this is that water promotes a temporarily increased circulation in the particular area of the diaphragm and stomach and thereby improves their contraction. Also, the absorption of cellular waste matter is accelerated, and muscle tone is improved.

The pack is applied for a minimum of three hours – but preferably at night and worn for the whole night. The immediate effect of the cold material on the skin and subcutaneous tissues is a contraction of the small blood vessels. This is followed very quickly by dilation, which is backed up by the deeper vessels, and general activity in the localized area is stimulated. After the first impact of cold, which should only last a few seconds, the pack should feel quite comfortable and gently warm. The frequency of application should be at least twice a week, regularly, for three weeks, at the beginning of the treatment.

To Make a Cold Pack

You will need four to six layers of cotton or linen material (old sheeting or towelling) 7 inches square.

A piece of old woollen material or flannelette 9 inches square.

A large towel folded lengthways to act as a binder.

3 large safety pins.

Method

Soak the cotton material in cold water, wring out very well until only damp, and smooth out any creases. Apply to upper abdomen, that is, just where the ribs divide, above and including the umbilicus (naval). Cover with the larger piece of blanket, making sure good contact with the skin is made, and bind on with the folded towel, firmly (but not too tightly). Pin in position; put on night wear and go to bed.

The pack should feel nicely warm – if not, two mistakes

might have been made. (1) The pack may not have been wrung out enough; (2) Contact may be poor and air may be entering between the skin and pack. If neither of these is true, then the vitality of the body is not yet strong enough to react properly and the pack should be discontinued, and tried later on in the treatment, say in two weeks time. It is important that the pack becomes warm and does not stay cold and clammy – it is only being effective if it warms up within the first ten minutes of application, otherwise, take it off.

Note: No waterproofing material should be used as this completely changes the effect of the pack, turning it into a poultice, which is not the effect wanted. When the pack is removed, after the three hours or in the morning as the case may be, the area should be washed with tepid water to remove traces of toxic material, eliminated through the skin.

There are several other ways in which water can be used therapeutically; One is always to finish a hot bath or shower with a cold splash. Begin with the legs and feet, as being the less sensitive parts, and work up to the arms, abdomen and back. This can be done with a sponge or with handfuls of water. Finish with a brisk rub down with a rough towel. The whole body will be glowing and alive.

SOME EXTRAS FOR TEMPORARY USE

Vitamin E: Wheatgerm oil capsules help in healing and in the better utilization of oxygen in the blood stream (100 IU strength, not more than three capsules daily). Discontinue after *six* weeks.

Herbal Tranquillizers: For the relief of tension, insomnia or general anxiety, a herbal tranquillizer, containing some of the B vitamins which help the nervous system may be used.

Tissue Salts: The biochemical trace elements which help to activate and balance bodily reactions are also important in the treatment of hiatus hernia. Calcium fluoride, which enhances elasticity, is particularly valuable in this case. These salts are obtainable at Health Food Stores and can be taken as directed. Neither the tissue salts nor the herbal tranquillizers should be taken for more than two months, and if necessary either or both could be resumed after an interval. But, the whole emphasis of natural treatment is to obviate the need for taking remedies, and to adjust the whole way of life to a healthy normality and balance.

4
Useful Recipes and Culinary Tips

Millet and Tomato Savoury
(to serve one)
2 oz (50g) millet
1 small tin tomatoes
1 clove of garlic (crushed)
2 teaspoonsful of mixed herbs
½ level teaspoonful of savory yeast extract.

Mix together in a steel pan and simmer gently until the millet has absorbed all the moisture. Stir fairly frequently. (Millet is similar to rice in cooking). Serve with vegetables.

Vinaigrette
2 tablespoonsful cider vinegar
1 tablespoonful sunflower seed oil
1 clove of garlic (crushed)
½ to 1 teaspoonful of honey
Any herb to flavour

Mix together.

Yogurt Mint Dressing

Simply chop one to two teaspoonsful of mint and add to the natural yogurt with a level teaspoonful of honey. Mix and use.

Stuffed Peppers – Red or Green

1 medium-sized pepper per person
1 tablespoonful brown rice per person
1 clove of garlic
2 teaspoonsful of mixed herbs
1 grated carrot per person
4 dried apricots per person

Cut off tops of peppers and remove the core and seeds – have an oven tin ready with half an inch of water to stand them in. Wash and part-boil the rice in salted water for 15 to 20 minutes, then drain and mix in garlic, herbs, carrots and apricots. Stuff this into the peppers and bake for 40-50 minutes at 375°F/190°C (Gas Mark 5) in the middle of the oven. Seasoning may be added sparingly.

Egg and Cheese Savoury

(to serve two)
2 eggs
$\frac{3}{4}$ pint (425ml) milk
1 teaspoonful mixed herbs
2 oz (50g) grated Cheddar cheese
Herbs (e.g. marjoram, rosemary etc.) optional

Beat the eggs well. Add milk and stir in the other ingredients. Put the mixture into a greased oven dish and stand this in a larger pan with half an inch of water. Bake at 350°F/180°C (Gas Mark 4) for 45 minutes or until set.

Home-made Muesli

1 lb (450g) oat, wheat or barley flakes (obtainable from Health Food Store)
4 oz (100g) raw cane sugar
4 oz (100g) raisins
4 oz (100g) chopped hazelnuts
2 oz (50g) dried milk powder
8 dried apricots, chopped small

Mix ingredients together ready for use and store in an air-tight tin or jar. Always eat with grated raw apple. It is better to soak each portion in water overnight, adding the apple in the morning.

Apple Crumble

(to serve 2)
2 cooking apples
1 dessertspoonful raw cane sugar
1 lemon, rind and juice
4 oz (100g) 100 per cent wholewheat flour
2 oz (50g) polyunsaturated margarine
1 tablespoonful raw cane sugar.

Core the apples and grate them together with skin into an oven dish. Add the juice and grated rind of the lemon, and the sugar. Mix gently. Top this mixture with the flour, sugar and margarine, mixed and rubbed together to form fine breadcrumbs. Press down slightly over the apple mixture. Bake at 400°F/200°C (Gas Mark 6) for 20-30 minutes.

Soya Savoury
(to serve 2)
1 small sliced onion
1 grated carrot
2 oz (50g) soya flakes
1 oz (25g) ground almonds
10 oz (275g) Cheddar cheese
1 tablespoonful sunflower seed oil
1 beaten egg
1 teaspoonful sage or mixed herbs
Water to mix, if necessary

Lightly fry the onion in the sunflower seed oil. Add to this the other dry ingredients, already mixed together in a bowl. Then add the egg, and water if necessary. This mixture can be cooked in three ways.

(1) Form into rissoles and fry in very little oil.
(2) Put the mixture into a greased oven dish to bake at 375°F/190°C (Gas Mark 5) for 25-35 minutes.
(3) Put the mixture into a greased basin. Cover this with greaseproof paper and steam for 30-40 minutes.

Chestnut Pudding
1 tin chestnut *purée*
1 teacup wholewheat breadcrumbs
1 small tin tomatoes
2 teaspoonsful mixed herbs
a little sea salt and black pepper (fresh ground)
2 tablespoonsful soya flour
1 small egg

Mix all the ingredients together (if too wet add more soya

flour), and put the mixture into a greased basin. Cover this securely with a cloth and steam it for one hour. Turn the pudding out onto a dish and serve. This dish looks good surrounded by a ring of mashed carrots, and can be eaten hot with vegetables or cold with a salad.

Making Juices Without a Juicer

This method could be used for root vegetables or any fruit that can be grated. You will need a soup plate or shallow dish, and a piece of gauze or muslin about twelve inches square, and a grater.

Arrange the muslin in the dish, grate the vegetable or fruit into it, then gather up the muslin carefully and squeeze out the juice from the pulp. Transfer the juice to a cup or mug and dilute it with one tablespoonful of water. Drink (sip) at once. (4 fl oz(100ml is the required amount.)

Carrot, beetroot and apple can be frequently used, and perhaps less frequently, because of their unusual taste, potato, swede and turnip.

Sprouting Seeds, Grains and Beans

Use a clear jar covered with gauze and secured by a rubber band. Put about a dessertspoonful of whatever seeds or grains you choose into the jar, and rinse well with cold water – no residue should be left in the jar. Put on the gauze lid. Each day rinse the seeds (it can be done through the lid without removing it) and drain well. Sprouts appear after three to six days. Allow them to grow to one or one-and-a-half inches, then remove from the jar and eat both the seeds and the sprouts. Begin the process again.

Some examples to try are:

Beans	*Seeds*	*Grains*
Adzuki	Alfalfa	Wheat
Mung	Mustard	Rye
Chickpeas	Cress	Barley
Soyabeans	Fennel	
Haricot	Sesame	
Black-eyed	Beet	
	Carrot	

Cooking Brown Rice

For $\frac{1}{2}$ lb (225g) of rice you will need: $1\frac{1}{2}$ pints (890ml) water; half a teaspoonful of sea salt; a teaspoonful of vegetable oil.

Wash the rice. Boil the water with the salt and oil. Add the rice and boil quickly for 25-35 minutes (it is better to have the rice chewy rather than mushy). Remove from the heat, turn the rice into a sieve and rinse with hot water. Drain well. Rice may be used with various accompaniments.

5.
Conclusion

The holistic approach to healing certainly requires time and application, if not dedication. However, the means of treatment are simple and they are safe.

Repressive treatment that is aimed mainly at relieving symptoms only prolongs the condition. In this case the patient may feel more comfortable, but nothing is being done to treat the cause, and most drug treatment produces side-effects of some sort. In addition, the body has to deal with the drugs whilst in a depleted or 'ill' state. This, in turn, increases the drain on vitality and further weakens the organism.

On the other hand, with natural treatment, after a short time patients are aware of a feeling of well-being and increased energy, even though there is still a lot to do, and some symptoms may persist. There is a feeling of 'rightness' about the regime which gives encouragement to persevere. Many patients have said that they had no idea how well they could feel, until they had tried natural healing.

The holistic approach is a way of life and not just aimed at curing conditions. By following this sensible plan, and then adopting it, with some adaptations, for the future, much ill-health will be prevented. It is certainly my sincere hope that readers will be encouraged to change their way of life, not just for the treatment of hiatus hernia but to improve their standard of health over all.

COMMONSENSE VEGETARIANISM

AN INTRODUCTION TO VEGETARIANISM GIVING AN EASY-TO-FOLLOW GUIDE ON PLANNING A WELL-BALANCED AND HEALTH-PROMOTING VEGETARIAN DIET

Harry Benjamin N.D. Written with the new convert and the interested non-vegetarian in mind, this book states clearly the facts and fictions of vegetarianism. It is also intended for those who have been vegetarians for a number of years but who nevertheless are ignorant of the basic principles of sound dietetics. *Includes:* The meat myth; Nature Cure and vegetarianism; Some popular misconceptions; Facts about animal and non-animal proteins; Preparing a healthful vegetarian diet.